The Herbal Zodiac:
Exploring the Medicinal Use of Herbs through Astrology

By: Tanya Smith

Chapter 1: *Introduction to Herbal Medicine and Astrology*

- Understanding the foundations of herbal medicine and its historical significance
- Introduction to astrology and its role in understanding the cosmic energy that influences our lives
- Highlighting the interconnectedness between herbs and astrology

Chapter 2: *The Elements and Their Corresponding Herbs*

- Exploring the characteristics and influences of the four elements: Fire, Earth, Air, and Water
- Identifying herbs corresponding to each element and their unique healing properties and planetary associations
- Understanding how the elements can impact our physical and emotional well-being

Chapter 3: *Herbal Remedies for the Zodiac Signs*

- Examining the twelve zodiac signs and their planetary rulerships
- Exploring the medicinal qualities of herbs that align with each zodiac sign
- Providing herbal remedies and recommendations for specific health concerns or imbalances associated with each zodiac sign

Chapter 4: *Planetary Influences and Herbal Healing*

- Investigating the seven classical planets and their influence on health and wellness
- Discovering the herbs associated with each planet and their healing properties
- Delving into planetary transits and their impact on our physical and emotional well-being

Chapter 5: *Planetary Associations with Body Systems and Organs*

- Exploring the connection between the planets and different body systems and organs
- Understanding how planetary transits and alignments can affect specific areas of our health
- Offering herbal remedies to support and harmonize the body systems associated with each planet

Chapter 6: *Creating Personalized Herbal Remedies with Astrology*

- Combining astrology and herbal medicine to create personalized healing blends
- Exploring astrological birth charts to identify individual health strengths and weaknesses
- Providing guidance on creating herbal formulations that align with an individual's unique astrological profile

Introduction

In this book, we embark on a fascinating journey that combines the ancient wisdom of herbal medicine with the guiding principles of astrology. By exploring the medicinal use of herbs in relation to the zodiac signs and planetary influences, we uncover a wealth of knowledge that can empower us to enhance our well-being and balance our mind, body, and spirit.

Through the pages of this book, I hope to inspire you to deepen your understanding of both herbal medicine and astrology. May you discover the transformative power of aligning with the natural rhythms of the universe, using herbs as allies to support your health and vitality.

Remember, this book serves as a guide, but ultimately, your intuition and inner wisdom should guide you in creating personalized herbal remedies that resonate with your unique needs and astrological influences.

Chapter 1

Herbal medicine and astrology are both ancient practices that have been used for centuries to provide healing, guidance, and wellbeing.

Herbal medicine, also known as herbalism or botanical medicine, is the use of plants and their extracts to treat various ailments and promote overall health. This practice dates back thousands of years and has been a significant part of traditional medicine systems in cultures all around the world. From ancient civilizations like Egypt, Greece, and China to indigenous cultures in North and South America, herbs have been revered for their medicinal properties and were often used in rituals and ceremonies.

The foundations of herbal medicine are based on the belief that plants contain vital energies and chemical compounds that can have profound effects on the body, mind, and spirit. Herbalists study different plants and their properties to create remedies, such as teas, tinctures, and salves, to support the body's natural healing processes.

Astrology, on the other hand, is the study of the movements and positions of celestial bodies, such as the sun, moon, planets, and stars, and their influence on human affairs and the natural world. It is an ancient practice that dates back to ancient Mesopotamia and has been embraced by various cultures and civilizations throughout history.

Astrologers believe that the positions of the celestial bodies at the time of a person's birth can provide insight into their personality traits, talents, and life path. They also believe that the planets and their energies can affect our emotions, relationships, and overall well-being. By studying the birth chart, which is a map of the sky at the time of birth, astrologers can provide guidance and predictions based on the planetary influences.

The connection between herbal medicine and astrology lies in their shared belief in the interconnectedness of all things in the natural world. Just as the planets and celestial bodies are believed to influence our lives, certain plants and herbs are associated with different zodiac signs and planets. These associations are based on the energetic properties and healing qualities attributed to the plants, which align with the characteristics of the zodiac signs and planetary influences.

For example, lavender is associated with the planet Mercury and the zodiac sign Virgo. Lavender is known for its calming and soothing properties, which align with the analytical and practical nature of Virgo. Similarly, St. John's Wort is associated with the sun and the zodiac sign Leo, as it is believed to enhance confidence and vitality, qualities often associated with the sun and the fiery energy of Leo.

By exploring the foundations of herbal medicine and astrology, we can deepen our understanding of the natural world and our place within it. We can tap into the healing properties of plants and herbs, and we can seek guidance and self-discovery through astrology. This integrated approach allows us to embrace the power of nature and the cosmos for our physical, mental, and spiritual well-being.

The foundations of herbal medicine can be traced back thousands of years to ancient civilizations and indigenous cultures around the world. These cultures recognized the power of plants and their ability to heal various ailments and promote overall health.

One of the earliest recorded examples of herbal medicine comes from ancient Mesopotamia, where clay tablets dating back to around 3000 BCE described the use of plants for medicinal purposes. The ancient Egyptians also extensively used herbal remedies, and their knowledge was recorded in the Ebers Papyrus, one of the oldest medical texts dating back to around 1550 BCE.

In ancient China, herbal medicine became an integral part of traditional Chinese medicine, with texts like the Huangdi Neijing (Yellow Emperor's Inner Canon) documenting the use of herbs to maintain health and treat diseases. Herbal medicine also played a significant role in ancient Greek and Roman civilizations, with Hippocrates, often referred to as the "father of medicine," emphasizing the healing properties of plants.

Indigenous cultures around the world, such as Native American tribes, Aboriginal Australians, and Maori people of New Zealand, have been using herbs and plants for healing purposes for generations. Their knowledge has been handed down through oral traditions and integrated into their respective traditional healing systems.

Herbal medicine methods and practices vary across different cultures, but they often involve the use of various parts of plants like the leaves, flowers, roots, bark, and seeds. These plant materials can be prepared and consumed in different ways, such as brewing teas, creating tinctures or extracts, making poultices or salves, and even through steam inhalation.

Historically, herbal medicine was often practiced by specialized healers or medicine men and women who possessed extensive knowledge of plants and their medicinal properties. These herbalists would gather, prepare, and administer remedies tailored to individual patients based on their specific symptoms and needs.

Throughout history, herbal medicine has gradually evolved and adapted, incorporating knowledge from different cultures and integrating with modern medical practices. Today, herbal medicine is recognized as a complementary and alternative medicine (CAM) practice, and many people seek out herbal remedies alongside conventional medical treatments for various ailments.

As more scientific research is conducted on the efficacy and safety of different herbs, we continue to uncover the therapeutic potential of plants and their active compounds. Herbal medicine remains a popular approach to promote holistic and natural healing, appreciating the power of nature and its ability to support our wellbeing.

Astrology is a belief system and practice that seeks to understand the influence of cosmic energy on human behavior and events. It is based on the notion that the positions and movements of celestial bodies, such as the sun, moon, planets, and stars, have a direct impact on our lives.

The origins of astrology can be traced back to ancient civilizations, including Mesopotamia, Egypt, India, and China. These cultures observed the patterns and movements of celestial bodies and developed complex systems to interpret their significance. Astrology was used for various purposes, such as predicting agricultural cycles, determining favorable times for certain activities, and providing guidance in personal matters.

In Western astrology, the zodiac is divided into twelve signs, each associated with a specific constellation and time of the year. These signs are believed to reflect particular character traits and tendencies that individuals born under them may possess. The position of the sun, moon, and planets at the time of a person's birth is mapped onto their natal chart, which serves as a snapshot of the cosmic energies present at that moment.

Astrologers analyze the natal chart to derive insights about a person's personality traits, strengths, weaknesses, and life events. They consider factors such as the placement of the sun, moon, and planets within the zodiac signs and houses, as well as their relationships to one another.

Astrology also incorporates the concept of planetary transits, which are the ongoing movements of celestial bodies in the sky. These transits are believed to influence different aspects of life and can indicate times of change, growth, challenges, or opportunities.

It is important to note that astrology does not claim to determine our fate or completely control our lives. Rather, it offers a framework for understanding the energies at play and provides a tool for self-reflection and personal growth. Astrology can help individuals gain insight into their strengths and weaknesses, make informed decisions, and navigate life's challenges.

While there is ongoing debate about the scientific validity of astrology, many people find value and meaning in its principles. Astrology continues to be practiced and studied by individuals who see it as a way to explore the interconnectedness between humans and the cosmos.

Ultimately, astrology offers a unique perspective on the cosmic energy that permeates our lives. It invites us to contemplate our place in the universe and seek harmony and alignment with the forces that shape our existence.

Herbs have long been associated with astrology and are believed to possess specific energies and properties that align with the characteristics of the zodiac signs and planetary influences. Here are some examples of the interconnectedness between herbs and astrology:

1. **Zodiac Sign Correspondences: Each zodiac sign is associated with certain herbs that are believed to resonate with their energy and characteristics.**

For example:

- **Aries**: Cayenne pepper for its fiery and energizing properties.

- **Taurus**: Basil for its grounding and comforting qualities.

- **Gemini**: Lavender for its calming and communication-enhancing effects.

- **Cancer**: Chamomile for its nurturing and soothing properties.

- **Leo**: Sunflower for its boldness and ability to radiate light.

- **Virgo**: Lemon balm for its purifying and organizing capabilities.

- **Libra**: Rose for its harmony-promoting and relationship-enhancing qualities.

- **Scorpio**: Patchouli for its sensual and transformative energies.

- **Sagittarius**: Sage for its wisdom-inspiring and protective properties.

- **Capricorn**: Comfrey for its grounding and stabilizing effects.

- **Aquarius**: Eucalyptus for its free-spirited and invigorating qualities.

- **Pisces**: Valerian for its dream-enhancing and intuitive properties.

2. **Planetary Influences: Astrology also associates herbs with specific planets and their corresponding energies.**

For example:

- **Sun**: Herbs such as chamomile, calendula, and St. John's wort, symbolizing vitality, confidence, and self-expression.

- **Moon**: Herbs like cucumber, jasmine, and mugwort, representing emotions, intuition, and nurturing.

- **Mercury**: Herbs such as peppermint, lavender, and fennel, associated with communication, intellect, and mental agility.

- **Venus**: Herbs like rose, yarrow, and hibiscus, signifying love, beauty, and harmony.

- **Mars**: Herbs such as ginger, nettle, and cayenne, symbolizing energy, passion, and courage.

- **Jupiter**: Herbs like cinnamon, ashwagandha, and dandelion, representing abundance, growth, and expansion.

- **Saturn**: Herbs such as comfrey, frankincense, and thyme, associated with discipline, structure, and grounding.

- **Uranus**: Herbs like lavender, lemongrass, and chamomile, signifying innovation, individuality, and awakening.

- **Neptune**: Herbs such as seaweed, white sage, and blue lotus, representing spirituality, dreams, and intuition.

- **Pluto**: Herbs like black cohosh, wormwood, and skullcap, symbolizing transformation, rebirth, and healing.

3. Ritual and Magic:

Astrology and herbs often intertwine in rituals and magical practices. People may use specific herbs during astrologically significant times or in combination with planetary alignments to enhance their intentions, manifestations, or spiritual practices. Examples include creating herbal baths, burning smudging herbs, making herbal sachets, or incorporating herbs into spellwork to align with specific astrological energies.

The interconnectedness between herbs and astrology provides individuals with a holistic approach to harnessing the energies of the cosmos and nature. Whether through personal rituals, herbal remedies, or simply incorporating herbs into daily life, many people find that combining astrology and herbs enhances their well-being and spiritual journey.

Chapter 2

The four elements—*Fire, Earth, Air, and Water*—are fundamental to astrology, as they are believed to represent different energies and qualities. Each element has corresponding herbs that align with its characteristics and influences:

1. <u>**Fire**</u>: The Fire element represents passion, energy, inspiration, and transformation. Corresponding herbs include:

- ***Cinnamon***: Known for its fiery and stimulating properties, cinnamon is associated with passion and creativity.
- ***Ginger***: With its warming and energizing qualities, ginger is linked to motivation and vitality.
- ***Rosemary***: Symbolizing courage and strength, rosemary is believed to kindle ambition and drive.
- ***Calendula***: This vibrant flower represents both fire and the sun, representing vitality and inner power.

2. <u>**Earth**</u>: The Earth element represents stability, grounding, abundance, and physical well-being. Corresponding herbs include:

- ***Patchouli***: Known for its grounding and stabilizing effects, patchouli promotes connection to the earth and fosters stability.
- ***Sage***: With its purifying and calming properties, sage is associated with wisdom, protection, and earthly abundance.
- ***Vetiver***: This earthy-scented grass is believed to bring a sense of rootedness and stability to the mind and body.
- ***Comfrey***: Often called "knitbone," comfrey is associated with healing and nourishing the physical body.

3. **Air**: The Air element represents intellect, communication, curiosity, and freedom. Corresponding herbs include:

- *Lavender*: Known for its calming and relaxing effects, lavender is often used for enhanced communication and mental clarity.
- *Peppermint*: With its invigorating and cooling properties, peppermint promotes mental alertness and focus.
- *Lemongrass*: Associated with mental clarity and inspiration, lemongrass is believed to stimulate the mind and encourage communication.
- *Eucalyptus*: With its fresh and uplifting scent, eucalyptus is used to clear the mind, promote mental flexibility, and enhance communication.

4. **Water**: The Water element represents emotions, intuition, fluidity, and healing. Corresponding herbs include:

- *Chamomile*: Known for its calming and soothing effects, chamomile promotes relaxation, emotional healing, and restful sleep.
- *Rose*: Associated with love and emotional balance, roses are often used for heart healing and to promote self-love.
- *Jasmine*: With its intoxicating scent, jasmine is believed to enhance intuition, sensuality, and emotional healing.
- *Ylang-Ylang*: Often used in aromatherapy for its calming and aphrodisiac properties, ylang-ylang promotes emotional release and harmony.

Using herbs aligned with the elements can bring balance and support to different aspects of our lives. Whether through herbal teas, essential oils, or incorporating herbs into rituals and ceremonies, incorporating the energy and properties of these herbs can help harness the elemental energies for personal growth and healing.

The elements—earth, air, fire, and water—are believed to influence various aspects of life, including our physical and emotional well-being. Each element is associated with specific qualities and characteristics, and understanding their impact can help us better understand ourselves and how to achieve balance and wellness.

1. Earth:

- *Healing Herbs*: Healing herbs associated with the earth element are generally grounding and nourishing. They provide stability, promote physical health, and support overall well-being. Examples include ashwagandha, ginger, ginseng, and marshmallow root.

- *Planetary Associations:* Earth is often associated with the planet Saturn, which represents structure, discipline, and grounding energy.

2. Air:

- *Healing Herbs*: Herbs associated with air are usually uplifting, refreshing, and promote mental clarity and communication. They are known for their ability to improve focus, relieve stress, and stimulate the mind. Examples include lavender, lemon balm, peppermint, and rosemary.

- *Planetary Associations*: Air is typically associated with the planets Mercury and Uranus. Mercury represents communication, intellect, and adaptability, while Uranus represents innovation and unexpected change.

3. Fire:

- *Healing Herbs*: Herbs associated with fire are energizing, invigorating, and can promote passion, motivation, and creativity. They are often used for digestion, circulation, and to ignite one's inner fire. Examples include cayenne pepper, cinnamon, garlic, and turmeric.

- *Planetary Associations*: Fire is commonly associated with the planets Mars and the Sun. Mars represents strength, courage, and assertiveness, while the Sun represents vitality, self-expression, and radiant energy.

4. Water:

- *Healing Herbs*: Herbs associated with water are calming, soothing, and have a strong connection to emotions, intuition, and healing on an emotional level. They are often used for relaxation, stress relief, and supporting the health of the kidneys and bladder. Examples include chamomile, jasmine, lavender, and passionflower.

- *Planetary Associations*: Water is associated with the planets Moon and Venus. The Moon represents emotions, intuition, and nurturing energy, while Venus represents love, beauty, and harmony.

**** It's important to note that herbal therapies should be approached with caution and under the guidance of a qualified professional. While herbs can offer valuable support, individual needs and sensitivities vary, and it's always important to consider any potential allergies, interactions with medications, or existing health conditions.**

Chapter 3

The twelve zodiac signs are each associated with specific planetary rulerships, which influence their characteristics, energies, and behaviors. Here is an overview of the zodiac signs and their planetary rulers:

Aries (March 21 - April 19):

- Ruled by Mars: Aries is known for its fiery and assertive energy, representing courage, passion, and initiation.

Taurus (April 20 - May 20):

- Ruled by Venus: Taurus embodies the sensual and earthy qualities of Venus, representing pleasure, stability, and material comfort.

Gemini (May 21 - June 20):

- Ruled by Mercury: Gemini is associated with the swift and communicative energy of Mercury, representing curiosity, intellect, and adaptability.

Cancer (June 21 - July 22):

- Ruled by the Moon: Cancer's emotional and nurturing nature is influenced by the Moon, symbolizing intuition, nurturing, and sensitivity.

Leo (July 23 - August 22):

- Ruled by the Sun: Leo's vibrant and charismatic energy is influenced by the Sun, representing vitality, self-expression, and leadership.

Virgo (August 23 - September 22):

- Ruled by Mercury: Virgo's analytical and detail-oriented nature is also influenced by Mercury, representing practicality, organization, and efficiency.

Libra (September 23 - October 22):

- Ruled by Venus: Libra embodies Venus' harmonious and diplomatic energy, symbolizing balance, beauty, and relationship-oriented qualities.

Scorpio (October 23 - November 21):

- Ruled by Pluto (traditional ruler) and Mars (modern ruler): Scorpio's intense and transformative energy is influenced by Pluto, representing power, depth, and regeneration.

Sagittarius (November 22 - December 21):

- Ruled by Jupiter: Sagittarius' expansive and freedom-loving nature is influenced by Jupiter, representing wisdom, growth, and exploration.

Capricorn (December 22 - January 19):

- Ruled by Saturn: Capricorn embodies Saturn's disciplined and ambitious energy, representing responsibility, structure, and long-term goals.

<u>Aquarius (January 20 - February 18):</u>

- Ruled by Uranus (modern ruler) and Saturn (traditional ruler): Aquarius' innovative and forward-thinking nature is influenced by Uranus, representing originality, independence, and humanitarian qualities.

<u>Pisces (February 19 - March 20):</u>

- Ruled by Neptune (modern ruler) and Jupiter (traditional ruler): Pisces' dreamy and compassionate energy is influenced by Neptune, symbolizing spirituality, creativity, and empathy.

The planetary rulerships provide insight into each zodiac sign's core nature and the energies that shape their personality traits, strengths, and areas of focus. However, it's essential to consider the entire birth chart and the interactions between different planets and signs for a comprehensive understanding of an individual's astrological makeup.

Here are some herbs associated with each zodiac sign and their medicinal qualities:

1. Aries:
   - Herb: Cayenne Pepper
   - Medicinal Qualities: Cayenne pepper is known for its warming properties, stimulating circulation, increasing energy, and promoting digestion. It is also used for its antibacterial and anti-inflammatory effects.

2. Taurus:
   - Herb: Chamomile
   - Medicinal Qualities: Chamomile is renowned for its calming and soothing effects. It is commonly used to relieve stress, anxiety, and promote relaxation. It is also known for its anti-inflammatory and digestive properties.

3. Gemini:
   - Herb: Peppermint
   - Medicinal Qualities: Peppermint is known for its cooling and refreshing properties. It helps to relieve indigestion, headaches, and nasal congestion. Peppermint also aids in mental clarity and improves focus.

4. Cancer:
   - Herb: Lemon Balm
   - Medicinal Qualities: Lemon balm has calming and uplifting properties. It is often used to alleviate anxiety, insomnia, and digestive issues. Lemon balm can also boost mood and promote relaxation.

5. Leo:
   - Herb: Rosemary
   - Medicinal Qualities: Rosemary has invigorating and stimulating properties. It is known for improving memory, concentration, and mental clarity. Rosemary also aids in digestion and is a potent antioxidant.

6. Virgo:
   - Herb: Lavender
   - Medicinal Qualities: Lavender is renowned for its calming and stress-relieving properties. It promotes relaxation, improves sleep quality, and reduces anxiety. Lavender is also a natural antiseptic and can be used topically for skin irritations.

7. Libra:
   - Herb: Passionflower
   - Medicinal Qualities: Passionflower has a calming effect and is often used to relieve anxiety, promote sound sleep, and reduce stress. It also helps to relax muscles and alleviate muscle tension.

8. Scorpio:
   - Herb: Sage
   - Medicinal Qualities: Sage has various medicinal properties, including antimicrobial, anti-inflammatory, and antioxidant effects. It is used to soothe sore throats, improve digestion, and relieve menopausal symptoms.

9. Sagittarius:
   - Herb: Ginseng
   - Medicinal Qualities: Ginseng is known for its energizing and adaptogenic properties. It helps increase stamina, improve cognitive function, and boost the immune system. Ginseng also aids in reducing stress and promoting overall well-being.

10. Capricorn:
   - Herb: Ashwagandha
   - Medicinal Qualities: Ashwagandha is an adaptogenic herb that helps the body manage stress, reduce anxiety, and improve energy levels. It also promotes balance, enhances cognitive function, and supports immune health.

11. Aquarius:
   - Herb: Echinacea
   - Medicinal Qualities: Echinacea is esteemed for its immune-boosting properties. It strengthens the immune system, aids in cold and flu prevention, and promotes overall wellness. Echinacea also has anti-inflammatory and antibacterial effects.

12. Pisces:
   - Herb: Passionflower
   - Medicinal Qualities: Passionflower has a calming effect and is often used to relieve anxiety, promote sound sleep, and reduce stress. It also helps to relax muscles and alleviate muscle tension.

Please note that while these herbs are associated with each zodiac sign, individual preferences and sensitivities may vary. It's always advisable to consult with a healthcare professional before incorporating any herbs or remedies into your lifestyle.

Planetary transits refer to the movement of planets as they traverse through the zodiac signs and interact with various aspects of our birth chart. These transits can have an impact on our physical and emotional well-being in several ways:

1. Energetic Shifts: Planetary transits can bring about shifts in energy, both individually and collectively. For example, a challenging transit from Mars may lead to increased feelings of agitation, irritability, or restlessness. On the other hand, a harmonious transit from Venus may bring about a sense of ease, pleasure, and emotional well-being.

2. Emotional Triggers: Certain transits can act as catalysts for emotional experiences. For instance, a transit from the Moon may heighten our sensitivity and emotional receptivity, potentially leading to heightened feelings or emotional reactions.

3. Physical Manifestations: Some transits can also influence our physical well-being. For instance, a transit from Saturn may highlight areas of the body that require attention, leading to increased awareness of physical discomfort or illness. Conversely, a beneficial transit from Jupiter may bring about a boost of vitality and overall well-being.

4. Personal Growth Opportunities: Challenging planetary transits can present opportunities for personal growth and transformation. They may bring unresolved emotions or patterns to the surface, prompting us to confront and work through them for our overall well-being.

5. Timing and Cycles: Planetary transits follow specific cycles and timing, which can affect our energy levels and overall well-being. Understanding these cycles can help us align our actions and make informed decisions regarding self-care during certain transits.

It is important to note that while planetary transits can provide insights into potential energetic influences, they should not be seen as deterministic or predictive of specific health outcomes. Each individual's birth chart, unique circumstances, and personal choices also play a significant role in shaping their well-being. Consulting with a professional astrologer or holistic practitioner can provide further guidance and insights into how planetary transits may impact your specific well-being.

Chapter 4

The classical planets, also known as the Seven Luminaries, include the Sun, Moon, Mercury, Venus, Mars, Jupiter, and Saturn. In astrology, each of these planets is believed to have a distinct influence on health and wellness based on their specific qualities and energies. Let's explore these influences:

Sun: The Sun represents vitality, energy, and overall well-being. Its influence is associated with the heart, spine, circulation, and immune system. A strong Sun is believed to promote good health, strength, and vitality.

Moon: The Moon is linked to emotional well-being and the body's fluids, including hormones and digestive juices. Its influence also extends to the breasts, stomach, and uterus. A balanced Moon is associated with emotional stability and proper fluid balance.

Mercury: Mercury governs communication, thinking, and the nervous system. It influences the brain, respiratory system, hands, and arms. A harmonious Mercury may contribute to clear thinking, effective communication, and good respiratory health.

Venus: Venus represents love, beauty, and pleasure. It influences the kidneys, throat, senses, and reproductive organs. Balanced Venus energy is associated with healthy kidney function, throat health, and harmonious relationships.

Mars: Mars is associated with energy, action, and drive. It influences the muscles, blood, adrenals, and the reproductive system in men. A balanced Mars fosters good muscular strength, healthy blood circulation, and balanced sex drive.

Jupiter: Jupiter signifies expansion, growth, and abundance. It influences the liver, gallbladder, metabolism, and general well-being. A well-placed Jupiter is associated with good digestion, liver health, and a robust metabolism.

Saturn: Saturn represents discipline, structure, and maturity. It influences the bones, teeth, skin, and the overall structural integrity of the body. A balanced Saturn is associated with strong bones, good dental health, and overall longevity.

*** It is important to note that these associations are based on astrological interpretations and are not scientifically proven. While astrology can provide insights into potential energetic influences, it is not a substitute for professional medical advice. Consultation with a healthcare professional is always recommended for any health concerns.*

Here are some herbs traditionally associated with each planet and their healing properties according to astrological traditions:

1. Sun: Calendula, St. John's Wort, Rosemary

- **Calendula**: Used for skin conditions, wound healing, and promoting overall vitality.
- **St. John's Wort**: Traditionally used for mood disorders, depression, and nerve-related pain.
- **Rosemary**: Known for its stimulating and invigorating properties, it is used to improve memory, digestion, and circulation.

2. Moon: Jasmine, White Willow, Clary Sage

- **Jasmine**: Used for its calming and mood-lifting properties, it is often used to relieve anxiety and insomnia.
- **White Willow**: Traditionally used as a natural analgesic to relieve pain and reduce inflammation.
- **Clary Sage**: Known for its hormone-balancing properties, it is used for menstrual discomfort, hormonal imbalances, and stress relief.

3. Mercury: Lavender, Peppermint, Eucalyptus

- **Lavender**: Known for its calming and balancing effects, it is used for stress relief, relaxation, and insomnia.
- **Peppermint**: Used to improve digestion, relieve headaches, and boost mental clarity and focus.
- **Eucalyptus**: Traditionally used for respiratory health, it has expectorant properties and is often used for congestion and respiratory infections.

4. Venus: Rose, Hibiscus, Damiana

- **Rose**: Known for its uplifting and heart-opening properties, it is used for emotional well-being and promoting self-love.
- **Hibiscus**: Traditionally used to support cardiovascular health and improve circulation.
- **Damiana**: Known as an aphrodisiac and mood enhancer, it is used for libido enhancement and overall well-being.

5. Mars: Cayenne, Ginger, Nettle

- **Cayenne**: Known for its warming and circulation-stimulating properties, it is used for pain relief and to improve digestion.
- **Ginger**: Used for its anti-inflammatory and digestive properties, it can help with nausea, indigestion, and joint pain.
- **Nettle**: Traditionally used for its diuretic and anti-inflammatory properties, it can be used for allergies, arthritis, and urinary issues.

6. Jupiter: Dandelion, Turmeric, Licorice

- **Dandelion**: Traditionally used for liver support and detoxification, it stimulates digestion and promotes healthy bile flow.
- **Turmeric**: Known for its anti-inflammatory properties, it is used for joint pain, digestive issues, and overall immune support.
- **Licorice**: Used for digestive health, adrenal support, and soothing inflamed mucous membranes.

7. Saturn: Comfrey, Horsetail, Sage

- **Comfrey**: Traditionally used for bone and tissue healing, it is used for fractures, sprains, and soothing inflamed tissues.

- **Horsetail**: Known for its high silica content, it supports healthy skin, hair, and nails. It may also support bone health.

- **Sage**: Traditionally used for its antiseptic and anti-inflammatory properties, it can be used for sore throat, gum health, and digestive issues.

*** Please note that while these herbs have been associated with specific planets, their healing properties and uses extend beyond astrological associations. Always consult with a healthcare professional or herbalist before using herbs for medicinal purposes, especially if you have any pre-existing health conditions or are taking medications.*

Planetary transits refer to the movements of planets as they travel through the zodiac signs and interact with different areas of our birth charts. These transits can have an impact on our physical and emotional well-being, as they can influence the energies and themes that are predominant at any given time. Here are some examples of how different planetary transits may affect us:

Sun Transits: The Sun represents our vitality, energy, and sense of self. During Sun transits, we may experience changes in our energy levels, mood, and overall well-being. For example, during a challenging aspect such as a square or opposition, we may feel more drained or encounter greater difficulties. On the other hand, during harmonious aspects like trines or sextiles, we may feel more energized and confident.

Moon Transits: The Moon represents our emotions, instincts, and inner world. Moon transits can greatly influence our emotional well-being and energy levels. For instance, a Full Moon may bring a surge of emotions to the surface, while a New Moon may offer a fresh start and a boost of motivation. Pay attention to the sign and aspects the Moon makes during its transit, as this can give you insights into what emotions and themes may be prevalent.

Mercury Transits: Mercury is associated with communication, thinking processes, and mental agility. During Mercury transits, we may notice changes in our mental focus, communication style, and ability to concentrate. For example, during a Mercury retrograde period, difficulties in communication and misunderstandings may arise. Conversely, during harmonious aspects, our thinking processes may become sharper, and our communication skills may improve.

Venus Transits: Venus represents love, relationships, beauty, and pleasure. During Venus transits, we may experience changes in our relationships, aesthetics, and sense of harmony. For instance, during a Venus retrograde, romantic relationships may encounter challenges or revisiting of past issues may occur. However, during positive aspects, there can be an increase in feelings of love, connection, and aesthetic appreciation.

Mars Transits: Mars governs energy, drive, and assertion. Mars transits can influence our motivation, physical energy levels, and ability to take assertive action. For example, during a Mars retrograde period, we may experience a decrease in motivation or encounter obstacles. But during harmonious aspects, our physical energy may increase, and we may find it easier to take decisive action towards our goals.

Jupiter Transits: Jupiter represents expansion, growth, and optimism. During Jupiter transits, we may experience an increase in opportunities, luck, and overall positivity. For instance, during a Jupiter transit to a favorable area of our chart, there may be opportunities for personal growth, success, and expansion. However, it's crucial to stay grounded and avoid overindulgence during these transits.

Saturn Transits: Saturn represents discipline, structure, and responsibility. Saturn transits often involve lessons, challenges, and tests of endurance. For example, during a Saturn transit to a particular area of our chart, we may encounter setbacks, limitations, or a need to take on more responsibilities. These periods require patience, perseverance, and a focus on long-term goals.

It's important to note that everyone's birth chart is unique, and the specific impact of a transit will depend on the individual's chart and personal circumstances. It's always beneficial to consult with an astrologer to gain a deeper understanding of how specific planetary transits may affect you personally.

Chapter 5

In astrology, different planets are associated with different body systems and organs based on the principle of correspondence or resonance. This connection is believed to reflect the energetic influence of the planets on our physical well-being. Here are some examples of these associations:

Sun: The Sun is associated with the heart, circulatory system, spine, and vitality. Its energy is said to influence our overall vitality, strength, and vitality.

Moon: The Moon is associated with the body's fluids, digestive system, reproductive system, and emotional well-being. Lunar transits may influence our emotional state, appetite, and fluid balance.

Mercury: Mercury is associated with the nervous system, brain, respiratory system, and communication. Its transits may influence our mental agility, cognitive functioning, and respiratory health.

Venus: Venus is associated with the kidneys, throat, senses, and reproductive organs. Its energy is said to influence our relationship with pleasure, beauty, and harmony.

Mars: Mars is associated with the muscles, energy levels, adrenal glands, and sex drive. Its energy is associated with action, passion, and motivation.

Jupiter: Jupiter is associated with the liver, gallbladder, metabolism, and expansion. Its energy is believed to bring about growth, abundance, and vitality.

Saturn: Saturn is associated with the bones, joints, teeth, skin, and structures of the body. Its energy is associated with discipline, responsibility, and the aging process.

Uranus: Uranus is associated with the nervous system, circulation, and electrical impulses in the body. Its energy is associated with change, innovation, and sudden disruptions.

Neptune: Neptune is associated with the immune system, lymphatic system, and connective tissues. Its energy is associated with spirituality, intuition, and transcendence.

Pluto: Pluto is associated with transformation, regeneration, and the hidden aspects of our being. Its energy is associated with deep, profound changes and the release of old patterns.

** It is important to note that these associations are based on astrological interpretation and are not scientifically proven. They provide a framework for understanding the potential energetic influences of the planets on our physical well-being. It is always advisable to seek professional medical advice for any health concerns and not solely rely on astrological associations.

Planetary transits and alignments can indeed have an impact on specific areas of our health. Astrology views the body, mind, and spirit as interconnected, and therefore, changes in energetic patterns can influence our physical health in various ways. Here are some examples of how specific planetary transits and alignments can affect different areas of our health:

1. Sun Transits: As the Sun represents our vitality and energy, its transits can impact our physical well-being. For instance, during a challenging Sun transit, we may experience a decrease in energy levels, feel exhausted, or encounter physical discomfort. Conversely, during harmonious Sun transits, we may feel more energized, experience improved physical health, and have a general sense of well-being.

2. Moon Transits: The Moon represents our emotions and instincts, and its transits can affect our mental and emotional well-being, which, in turn, can influence our physical health. For example, during a particularly intense Moon transit, such as a lunar eclipse, we may experience heightened emotions, which can impact our stress levels and potentially manifest as physical symptoms like headaches or digestive issues. Conversely, during a soothing Moon transit, we may feel more emotionally balanced, leading to improved physical health.

3. Mars Transits: Mars is associated with energy, drive, and physical activity. During Mars transits, there can be an increase or decrease in physical energy levels, which can affect our overall health. For instance, during a challenging Mars transit, we may feel drained, fatigued, or encounter health issues related to inflammation or physical strain. However, during harmonious Mars transits, we may experience increased physical vitality and find it easier to engage in exercise and physical activities that promote good health.

4. Saturn Transits: Saturn is often associated with structure, discipline, and limitations. During Saturn transits, we may encounter lessons and challenges that can impact our physical health. For example, a Saturn transit to a specific area of our chart may bring about health issues or require us to adopt healthier lifestyle habits. Saturn's influence encourages us to take responsibility for our well-being and make necessary changes to improve our health and overall quality of life.

5. <u>Neptune Transits:</u> Neptune symbolizes spirituality, dreams, and transcendence. Its transits can affect our overall well-being, including our physical health. During Neptune transits, we may experience increased sensitivity, which can manifest in various ways, such as feeling drained, experiencing unexplained symptoms, or encountering challenges in accurately diagnosing certain health issues. It's important to practice self-care, grounding techniques, and seek medical advice when necessary during Neptune transits.

***It's worth noting that these examples are generalized, and individual experiences can vary depending on the specific aspects and placements in a person's birth chart. Additionally, it's crucial to understand that while astrology can provide insights and potential influences, it should not replace professional medical advice or treatment. If you have specific health concerns, it's always best to consult with a healthcare professional.*

While astrology can provide insights into how planetary transits may influence our health, it's important to approach herbal remedies with caution. While herbs can offer support and promote balance within our body systems, it's crucial to consult with a qualified herbalist or healthcare professional before incorporating them into your wellness routine. Here are some general suggestions for herbal remedies that may support and harmonize the body systems associated with each planet:

1. Sun (Vitality, Energy, Circulation): Herbs that are known to have energizing and circulatory properties, such as ginseng, ginger, cayenne pepper, and rosemary, may be beneficial in promoting overall vitality and supporting the cardiovascular system.

2. Moon (Emotions, Digestion, Hormonal Balance): Calming and nurturing herbs like chamomile, lavender, passionflower, and peppermint can help soothe the nervous system, promote healthy digestion, and support hormonal balance.

3. Mars (Physical Energy, Muscular Health): Herbs with stimulant properties, such as ginkgo biloba, gotu kola, ashwagandha, and rhodiola, may assist in boosting physical energy levels and supporting muscular health.

4. Saturn (Structural Health, Detoxification): Herbs that support bone, joint, and structural health, like turmeric, milk thistle, dandelion root, and nettle, can help facilitate detoxification and promote overall structural well-being.

5. Neptune (Sensitivity, Immunity, Rejuvenation): Adaptogenic herbs such as holy basil, astragalus, reishi mushroom, and schisandra can strengthen the immune system, support rejuvenation, and help manage sensitivity.

*** It's important to remember that everyone's needs are unique, and what works for one person may not work for another. Different body types, existing conditions, and sensitivities should all be taken into account when considering herbal remedies. It's highly recommended that you consult with a qualified herbalist or healthcare professional to ensure the herbs you choose are safe and suitable for you.*

Chapter 6

Combining astrology and herbal medicine to create personalized healing blends can be a fascinating and powerful way to support your health and well-being. Here's a step-by-step process to help you get started:

Consult with an Herbalist or Holistic Practitioner: Work with a qualified herbalist or holistic practitioner who is knowledgeable about both astrology and herbal medicine. They can guide you through the process and help you select the most appropriate herbs based on your astrological chart, individual needs, and any existing health conditions.

Interpret your Astrological Chart: Your astrological chart provides insights into your unique strengths, challenges, and potential health imbalances. Focus on the planetary placements and aspects that may influence your health, such as the Sun, Moon, Ascendant, and any planets that are prominently placed or in challenging aspects.

Match Planetary Energies with Herbs: Research and identify herbs that correspond to the planetary energies you want to balance or enhance. Consider both the traditional associations between herbs and planets, as well as the specific properties and actions of the herbs themselves. Look for herbs that align with both the astrological significance and your health goals.

Select Complementary Herbs: Explore combinations of herbs that work well together to create synergetic effects. For example, if you're focusing on Mars energy for physical energy and muscular health, you could combine stimulating herbs like ginkgo biloba and rhodiola with nourishing herbs like nettle and ashwagandha.

Consider Dosages and Preparations: Determine the appropriate dosages and preparations for each herb in your blend. This will depend on various factors, including the intended use, the herb's potency, and your individual needs. Your herbalist or holistic practitioner can guide you in finding the right balance and form, whether it's tinctures, teas, capsules, or topical applications.

Monitor and Adjust: As you start using your personalized herbal blend, pay attention to how your body responds. Monitor any changes in your energy levels, mood, digestion, or overall well-being. If needed, consult with your herbalist or holistic practitioner to make adjustments to the blend or dosages based on your feedback.

Regular Check-ins: Schedule regular check-ins with your herbalist or holistic practitioner to assess your progress, discuss any concerns or changes in your health, and make appropriate modifications to your herbal blend if necessary.

***** Remember, herbal medicine is a holistic approach that works best when combined with a healthy lifestyle, proper nutrition, exercise, and any other necessary conventional medical treatments. Always seek guidance from a qualified professional to ensure the herbs you choose are safe and appropriate for your unique needs.***

Exploring astrological birth charts can offer valuable insights into a person's individual health strengths and weaknesses. Here are some steps to help you identify these aspects:

1. Obtain a Copy of Your Birth Chart: You'll need to have your accurate date, time, and place of birth to generate your birth chart. There are various online resources and astrological software that can help you with this.

2. Identify Key Health-Related Planets: Look at the placements of certain planets in your birth chart that are associated with health and well-being. Some important planets to consider include the Sun, Moon, Ascendant (rising sign), and the sixth house, which is traditionally associated with health.

3. Analyze the Sign Placements: Pay attention to the zodiac signs in which these health-related planets are located. Each sign has unique characteristics and influences how the energy of the planet is expressed. Some signs may naturally enhance or challenge health-related energies.

4. Consider Planetary Aspects: Examine the aspects between the health-related planets and other planets in your birth chart. Aspects describe the angles formed between planets and can indicate how different energies interact and influence one another. Challenging aspects may indicate potential health vulnerabilities or imbalances.

5. Look for Patterns and Themes: Notice any patterns or recurring themes in your birth chart related to health. For example, if you have several planets in earth signs, it may suggest a grounded and practical approach to health. Conversely, if you have many planets in fire signs, it could indicate a need for balancing excess energy or tempering inflammation.

6. Consult with an Astrologer: Consider seeking guidance from a professional astrologer who specializes in medical or health astrology. They can help you interpret your birth chart and provide specific insights into your individual health strengths and weaknesses, as well as potential remedies or preventive measures.

*** Remember that astrology is not a substitute for professional medical advice, diagnosis, or treatment. It is a complementary tool that can provide insights and guidance. Always consult with a healthcare professional for any health concerns or issues you may have.*

Creating herbal formulations that align with an individual's astrological profile can be a creative and personalized approach to herbal medicine. Here's a step-by-step guide to help you get started:

1. Understand the Astrological Elements: Each zodiac sign is associated with one of four elements: fire, earth, air, or water. These elements represent different energetic qualities and can guide your herbal formulation. Fire signs tend to be energetic and passionate, earth signs grounded and practical, air signs intellectual and communicative, and water signs emotional and intuitive.

2. Consider Planetary Rulerships: Each zodiac sign is ruled by a specific planet, which can offer further insights into an individual's health and well-being. For example, Mars rules Aries and is associated with energy and vitality, while Venus rules Taurus and is connected to pleasure and sensuality. Understanding these planetary rulerships can guide your herbal choices.

3. Research Herbal Associations: Explore the medicinal properties and energetics of different herbs to find ones that align with the astrological elements and rulerships. For example, herbs like ginger and cayenne (fire), dandelion and ashwagandha (earth), lavender and peppermint (air), and chamomile and rose (water) can be considered based on their elemental affiliations.

4. Consider Traditional Medicinal Systems: Explore traditional medicinal systems like Ayurveda and Traditional Chinese Medicine (TCM), which also incorporate elemental and energetic principles. These systems offer extensive herbal knowledge and may provide additional guidance for creating personalized formulations based on an individual's elemental and astrological constitution.

5. Customize the Formulation: Once you have identified herbs that align with the individual's astrological profile, create a customized herbal formulation. This can be a combination of teas, tinctures, capsules, or topical preparations, depending on the specific health concerns or goals.

6. Consult with an Herbalist: If you are unfamiliar with herbal medicine or want a professional opinion, consider consulting with a qualified herbalist or holistic practitioner with knowledge in astrology and herbalism. They can provide personalized guidance based on your astrological profile and health needs.

*** Remember that herbal formulations are not a substitute for professional medical advice or treatment. Always consult with a healthcare professional before starting any herbal regimen, especially if you have specific health concerns or are taking medications.*

Author Notes

*** Exploring the medicinal use of herbs through astrology can be a unique and personalized approach to herbal medicine. By understanding an individual's astrological profile, including their elemental affiliations and planetary rulerships, herbal formulations can be tailored to support their specific health and well-being. Incorporating traditional medicinal systems and consulting with herbal experts can further enhance the formulation process. However, it's important to remember that astrology-based herbal formulations should be used as a complementary approach and not as a replacement for professional medical advice. Consulting with a healthcare professional is always recommended, especially for individuals with specific health concerns or taking medications.*

In this book, we have explored the fascinating intersection of herbal medicine and astrology. By harnessing the healing properties of herbs and understanding their correlations to the zodiac signs and planetary influences, we can nurture our well-being in a profound and holistic way.

May your journey into the medicinal use of herbs and astrology be filled with discovery, healing, and self-empowerment. May you find harmony and balance in your mind, body, and spirit by embracing the wisdom of these ancient practices.

Glossary:

1. Astrology: A belief system that connects celestial movements and positions with human events and characteristics.

2. Medicinal Herbs: Plants that have been traditionally used for their healing properties, often for medicinal purposes.

3. Zodiac Signs: Twelve astrological divisions of the celestial belt, representing specific personality traits and characteristics.

4. Planets: Celestial bodies that have significant astrological influences on different aspects of human life.

5. Planetary Rulerships: The association of certain herbs and plants with specific planets based on their astrological properties.

6. Sun Sign: The zodiac sign in which the sun is situated at the time of one's birth, believed to influence personality traits and health.

7. Moon Sign: The zodiac sign in which the moon is positioned at the time of one's birth, believed to affect emotions and well-being.

8. Ascendant (Rising Sign): The zodiac sign that is rising in the eastern horizon at the time of one's birth, influencing appearance and demeanor.

9. Herbal Medicine: The practice of utilizing herbs and plants for their therapeutic benefits.

10. Astrological Correspondences: The connections between specific herbs and their astrological attributes, such as ruling planet, element, and zodiac sign.

11. Elemental Associations: The connection of herbs with one of the four elements (fire, earth, air, water) based on their characteristics and actions.

12. Herbal Energetics: The concept that herbs have specific energetic qualities that can balance and restore the body and mind.

13. Planetary Herbalism: The use of planetary associations in herbal medicine to enhance the effectiveness of herbal remedies.

14. Herbal Formulations: The creation of herbal remedies by combining multiple herbs to address specific health concerns.

15. Astrological Timing: The consideration of astrological influences when choosing the appropriate time to harvest, prepare, or administer herbal remedies.

16. Natal Chart: A graphical representation of the position of celestial bodies at the time of one's birth, used in astrology to analyze and interpret personality traits and health tendencies.

17. Doctrine of Signatures: The belief that the physical characteristics of plants reveal their medicinal properties.

18. Herbal Infusions: Herbal preparations made by steeping herbs in hot water to extract their medicinal properties.

19. Tincture: A concentrated herbal extract, usually made by soaking herbs in alcohol or another solvent to extract their active constituents.

20. Herbal Poultice: A topical application of herbs, usually made by crushing or grinding fresh or dried herbs and applying them to the skin for localized healing.

While there are limited scientific studies on the medicinal use of herbs through astrology, there are numerous books and resources that explore the subject from a holistic and metaphysical perspective. It's important to note that the information provided in these sources should be approached with an open mind and critical thinking. Here are some recommended resources:

1. "The Complete Guide to Herbal Medicines" by Charles W. Fetrow and Juan R. Avila

   - This comprehensive guide provides in-depth information on medicinal herbs, including their traditional uses and scientific research.

2. "The Healing Power of Planetary Metals in Anthroposophic and Hermetic Medicine" by Dr. Jörg Wichmann

   - This book explores the use of planetary metals in herbal medicine, taking into account astrological correspondences.

3. "Medical Astrology" by Eileen Nauman

   - This book examines the connection between astrology and health, including the use of herbs and natural remedies based on astrological influences.

4. "Astrological Herbalism: Plant Medicine for Aries Through Virgo" by William Morris and Charles Obert

   - This book provides insights into the use of herbal medicine based on astrological characteristics of zodiac signs.

5. "The Herbs of the Northern Shaman" by Raven Kaldera

   - This book offers a cross-cultural perspective on herbal medicine, including astrological and metaphysical associations.

*** Additionally, online resources, such as blogs and forums dedicated to astrology, herbalism, and holistic healing, may provide valuable insights and personal experiences shared by practitioners and enthusiasts. It's important to approach these sources critically and consult with a qualified healthcare professional before using any herbs or herbal remedies.*